HOW TO DO YOGA FOR SENIORS

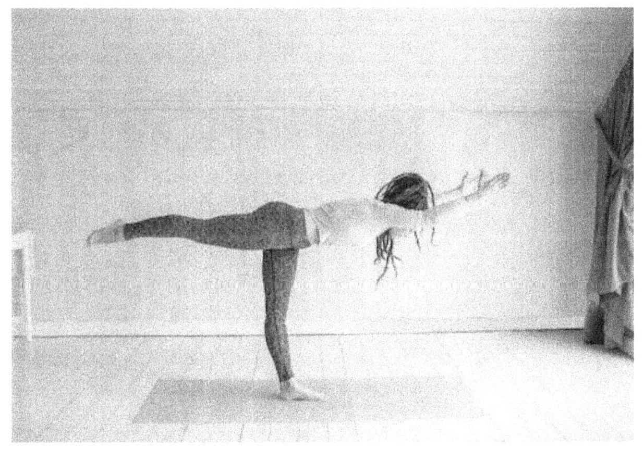

DR. VICKIE STOCK

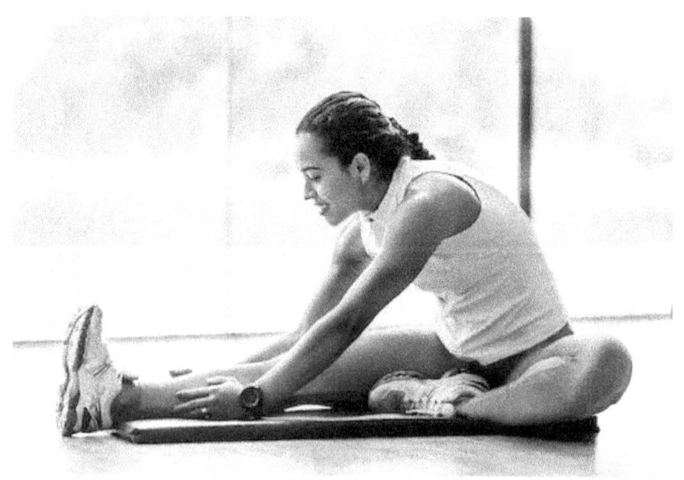

TABLE OF CONTENT

INTRODUCTION

Yoga, an ancient practice rooted in holistic well-being, offers a unique and gentle approach to fostering health and vitality among seniors. In this guide, we embark on a journey tailored specifically for older adults, exploring the transformative power of yoga for both the body and mind.

As we age, maintaining flexibility, strength, and mental acuity becomes increasingly essential. Yoga, with its gentle postures, mindful breathing, and meditative aspects, emerges as a beacon of rejuvenation.

Unlike strenuous exercises, yoga caters to the unique needs of seniors, promoting physical resilience and mental serenity without excessive strain.

Our exploration begins by unraveling the myriad benefits that yoga unfolds for seniors. From enhancing flexibility and balance to mitigating the impact of chronic conditions, yoga stands as a versatile tool for overall well-being.

However, safety is paramount, and we delve into considerations and precautions to ensure a secure and enjoyable practice.

Building a foundation, we set realistic goals, understanding that the beauty of yoga lies not in achieving perfection but in embracing progress. Each individual is encouraged to embark on a personal journey, discovering the transformative potential of yoga at their own pace.

In subsequent chapters, we guide seniors through gentle yoga poses, emphasizing seated and standing postures tailored to enhance flexibility, strength, and balance. Mindfulness and relaxation techniques take center stage, introducing meditation and breathing exercises to foster mental clarity and tranquility.

This guide isn't merely a manual; it's an invitation to seniors to carve out moments of serenity, rediscovering a sense of harmony through the practice of yoga.

Together, we embark on a path that celebrates the union of mind, body, and spirit, fostering a healthier, more vibrant life for seniors through the timeless art of yoga.

CHAPTER ONE

Types of **yoga** for seniors

Yoga for seniors encompasses a diverse range of practices that cater to varying abilities, preferences, and health conditions.

These specialized types of yoga offer tailored approaches to accommodate the unique needs of seniors, promoting physical well-being, mental clarity, and a sense of community. Here are some notable types of yoga for seniors:

1. Chair Yoga:

Chair yoga is a gentle form of yoga that allows seniors to practice while seated or using a chair for support. This type of yoga is particularly beneficial for individuals with limited mobility, joint issues, or balance concerns.

Chair yoga incorporates modified poses and stretches, making it accessible and safe for seniors while promoting flexibility and relaxation.

2. Gentle Yoga:

Gentle yoga is characterized by slow and mindful movements, emphasizing proper alignment and breath awareness. This type of yoga is well-suited for seniors who prefer a slower pace and a more relaxed approach.

Gentle yoga classes often include modifications to accommodate individual needs, making it ideal for those with varying fitness levels.

3. Restorative Yoga:

Restorative yoga focuses on deep relaxation and stress reduction. In restorative yoga, props such as blankets, bolsters, and cushions are used to support the body in comfortable and passive poses.

This type of yoga promotes a profound sense of calmness, making it beneficial for seniors seeking to release tension and cultivate a state of deep relaxation.

4. Hatha Yoga:

Hatha yoga is a foundational style that encompasses a broad range of physical postures and breathing exercises. It provides a well-rounded practice suitable for seniors, emphasizing balance, strength, and flexibility. Hatha yoga classes can be adapted to meet the needs of seniors, with instructors offering modifications for individual comfort and safety.

5. Iyengar Yoga:

Iyengar yoga places a strong emphasis on alignment and precision in poses. Props such as belts, blocks, and straps are commonly used to help practitioners achieve optimal alignment.

This style is suitable for seniors looking to refine their postures and build strength gradually. Iyengar yoga's meticulous approach ensures that seniors can practice safely with a focus on precision.

6. Kundalini Yoga:

Kundalini yoga combines physical postures, breathwork, and meditation to enhance spiritual and physical well-being.

While Kundalini yoga can be dynamic, it can also be adapted for seniors with gentler movements and modifications. The incorporation of breathwork and meditation makes

Kundalini yoga suitable for seniors seeking a holistic practice that nurtures both body and mind.

7. Yin Yoga:

Yin yoga focuses on long-held, passive poses targeting connective tissues. This style enhances flexibility and joint mobility, making it beneficial for seniors dealing with stiffness or reduced range of motion. Yin yoga encourages practitioners to find comfort in stillness, promoting relaxation and a sense of inner calm.

When seniors explore these types of yoga, they gain the flexibility to choose practices that align with their physical abilities and personal preferences.

Whether seated in a chair, moving gently through poses, or enjoying the restorative benefits of a prop-supported session, seniors can find a yoga style that supports their journey to enhanced well-being and mindful aging.

Yoga equipments for seniors

Yoga equipment for seniors plays a vital role in ensuring a safe, comfortable, and accessible practice that caters to their unique needs and physical conditions.

The right yoga props and accessories provide support, aid in stability, and enhance the overall experience. Here are essential yoga equipments for seniors:

1. Yoga Mat:

A high-quality, non-slip yoga mat is a fundamental accessory for seniors. The mat provides a stable surface for poses, reducing the risk of slips and falls.

Look for mats with adequate cushioning to support joints and ensure a comfortable practice. Non-toxic, eco-friendly materials are recommended for seniors with sensitivities.

2. Yoga Blocks:

Yoga blocks offer valuable support, helping seniors maintain proper alignment and ease into poses. These lightweight props can be placed under the hands, feet, or buttocks to adapt poses according to individual flexibility and comfort levels. Blocks are especially useful for seniors with limited range of motion or stiffness.

3. Yoga Straps:

Yoga straps assist in achieving proper alignment and stretching safely.

Seniors can use straps to extend their reach in various poses, enhancing flexibility without strain. The adjustable nature of yoga straps accommodates different body sizes and levels of flexibility, making them an excellent tool for seniors looking to improve their range of motion.

4. Chair:

A sturdy chair serves as a versatile prop for chair yoga, a modified practice that accommodates seniors with limited mobility or those who prefer seated exercises. Chairs provide support during standing poses, balance work, and stretches. Chair yoga is accessible and beneficial for seniors with varying physical abilities.

5. Bolsters:

Bolsters are large, firm cushions that enhance relaxation and comfort during restorative yoga poses. Seniors can use bolsters to support the spine, knees, or neck, promoting a sense of ease during gentle stretches. Bolsters are particularly valuable for seniors seeking a restful and rejuvenating practice.

6. Blankets:

Soft blankets offer additional comfort and support, especially during seated or reclining poses. Seniors can use blankets to cushion the joints and create a cozy environment for relaxation. Additionally, folded blankets can provide extra height or padding in seated poses, promoting proper alignment.

7. Cushions and Meditation Pillows:

Comfortable cushions or meditation pillows are essential for seated meditation and breathing exercises. These props alleviate pressure on the hips and knees, making it easier for seniors to maintain a comfortable and upright posture during meditation sessions.

8. Non-Slip Socks or Grippy Socks:

Non-slip socks with grippy soles provide seniors with additional traction, especially if practicing on hardwood or smooth surfaces.

These socks enhance stability and reduce the risk of slipping during standing poses or transitions.

9. Eye Pillow:

An eye pillow can be used during relaxation poses to block out light and promote a sense of calm. The gentle pressure from the eye pillow can also help alleviate tension around the eyes and forehead, enhancing the relaxation response.

10. Water Bottle:

Staying hydrated is crucial during any yoga practice. Seniors should keep a water bottle within reach to ensure they stay hydrated throughout the session. Proper hydration supports joint health and overall well-being.

Ensuring that seniors have access to these yoga props and accessories enables them to tailor their practice to their specific needs, promoting a safe, enjoyable, and effective yoga experience.

The right equipment empowers seniors to explore the benefits of yoga at their own pace while prioritizing comfort and well-being.

Understanding the Benefits of Yoga for Older Adults

Yoga, with its roots deeply embedded in ancient traditions, emerges as a beacon of holistic well-being, offering a plethora of benefits uniquely tailored to the needs of older adults. As we age, maintaining physical health, mental clarity, and emotional balance becomes paramount, and yoga presents itself as a gentle yet powerful tool for achieving these goals.

One of the primary benefits of yoga for seniors lies in its ability to enhance flexibility and mobility. The gentle stretching and range-of-motion exercises inherent in yoga postures contribute to increased flexibility, helping to alleviate stiffness in joints and muscles.

Improved flexibility not only enhances day-to-day activities but also reduces the risk of injury and promotes an overall sense of physical comfort.

Balance is another crucial aspect of well-being that tends to decline with age. Yoga, especially poses that focus on stability and grounding, helps seniors improve balance and coordination.

These practices are particularly valuable in preventing falls, a significant concern for older adults, and fostering a sense of confidence in everyday movements.

Moreover, the meditative and mindfulness components of yoga hold immense benefits for the mental health of seniors. Regular practice has been shown to reduce stress, anxiety, and depression, offering a sanctuary for calming the mind amidst life's challenges.

Mindfulness techniques incorporated into yoga, such as focused breathing and guided meditation, provide a mental respite, promoting a positive outlook and emotional resilience.

As the body ages, so does the risk of chronic conditions such as arthritis, osteoporosis, and cardiovascular issues. Yoga serves as a gentle yet effective ally in managing these conditions.

Specific postures and movements can help alleviate symptoms, improve joint function, and enhance cardiovascular health. It's a proactive approach to wellness that empowers seniors to take charge of their health and mitigate the impact of chronic conditions.

Social connection is integral to mental well-being, and yoga provides a unique opportunity for older adults to engage in a supportive community.

Whether practiced individually at home or in a group setting, yoga fosters a sense of belonging and shared purpose, creating a supportive environment for seniors to connect, share experiences, and build relationships.

Yoga for older adults transcends the physical postures; it becomes a comprehensive approach to enhancing the quality of life. By embracing the benefits of yoga, seniors embark on a journey of self-discovery, fostering physical resilience, mental serenity, and a renewed sense of vitality.

It's an invitation to experience the transformative power of yoga, promoting a fulfilling and empowered journey through the golden years.

Safety Considerations and Precautions in Senior Yoga Practice

Embarking on a yoga journey in the golden years is a commendable step towards holistic well-being, but ensuring safety is paramount to derive maximum benefits from the practice. Seniors, with their unique physical considerations, should approach yoga with mindfulness and an understanding of their individual needs.

Here, we delve into essential safety considerations and precautions to create a secure and enjoyable yoga experience for older adults.

First and foremost, it's imperative for seniors to consult with their healthcare provider before commencing a yoga practice. This ensures that any pre-existing health conditions or concerns are taken into account, and the yoga routine can be tailored to individual needs.

A collaborative approach between healthcare professionals and yoga instructors can contribute significantly to a safe and effective practice.

Adaptability is key. Yoga poses can be modified to accommodate different fitness levels and physical abilities. Seniors should feel empowered to communicate openly with their instructors about any discomfort or challenges they may be facing. A skilled yoga instructor with experience in teaching older adults can provide appropriate modifications and alternatives, ensuring that each participant can engage in the practice comfortably and safely.

Balance poses, while beneficial for improving stability, should be approached with caution. Seniors can use props such as chairs or walls for support during standing poses to minimize the risk of falls.

Additionally, incorporating seated or reclined variations of poses can provide the same benefits without putting undue stress on joints or compromising stability.

Joint health is a priority for older adults, and awareness of any limitations is crucial. Seniors should practice within a pain-free range of motion, avoiding overstretching or straining joints.

Gentle movements and gradual progression are key elements of a safe yoga practice, allowing the body to adapt and build strength over time.

Breathing exercises, a fundamental aspect of yoga, should be practiced with mindfulness. Seniors with respiratory conditions should consult their healthcare provider to ensure that specific breathing techniques align with their health needs. Modified breathwork can be incorporated to enhance lung capacity without causing strain.

Hydration is often overlooked but is essential, especially for seniors engaging in physical activity. Staying well-hydrated supports joint function and overall bodily functions, contributing to a safer and more comfortable yoga practice.

Creating a safe environment is equally important. Seniors should practice in a well-lit, clutter-free space, and non-slip mats can be employed to prevent slips or falls. Additionally, a gradual warm-up before the yoga session helps prepare muscles and joints for movement, reducing the risk of injury.

Embracing yoga in later years is a wonderful endeavor, but prioritizing safety considerations and taking necessary precautions ensures a positive and enriching experience.

By fostering open communication with healthcare professionals and instructors, practicing within individual abilities, and creating a safe physical space, seniors can embark on a yoga journey that promotes well-being, vitality, and a profound sense of self-care.

Setting Realistic Goals for Seniors in Yoga Practice

Embarking on a yoga journey in the golden years brings a myriad of physical and mental benefits, and setting realistic goals is a key element to ensure a fulfilling and sustainable practice.

For seniors, the essence of goal-setting in yoga lies in cultivating self-awareness, embracing individual differences, and recognizing that progress is a deeply personal and ongoing journey.

The first step in establishing realistic goals for seniors involves acknowledging and accepting the body's current state. Each individual enters the practice with a unique set of abilities, challenges, and health considerations.

Realistic goals, therefore, are rooted in an understanding of one's own physical condition, limitations, and aspirations. This self-awareness forms the foundation upon which a personalized and attainable yoga journey is built.

One primary goal for many seniors is to enhance flexibility and mobility. However, it's crucial to approach this with patience and gradual progression.

Setting a realistic target, such as improving the range of motion in a specific joint or achieving a comfortable seated position, allows seniors to experience tangible progress without undue strain.

Strength and balance are integral aspects of a senior's well-being, especially in the context of preventing falls and maintaining independence.

Realistic goals in these areas might involve mastering foundational standing poses, gradually increasing the duration of balance postures, or improving overall muscle tone.

These goals, when approached with mindfulness, contribute to a sense of accomplishment and enhanced physical resilience.

Mental well-being is equally important, and yoga provides a holistic platform for fostering emotional balance and tranquility. Seniors might set goals related to stress reduction, improved focus, or incorporating mindfulness into daily life. Realistic expectations in this realm involve recognizing the fluctuations of the mind and celebrating small victories in achieving a more serene and centered state.

Consistency is key in yoga, and seniors should set realistic goals regarding the frequency and duration of their practice. Rather than aiming for extensive sessions daily, establishing a manageable routine—perhaps a few shorter sessions per week—ensures that the practice remains enjoyable and sustainable over the long term.

Additionally, seniors can set goals related to the exploration of different yoga styles and practices. Trying a variety of poses, breathing techniques, and meditation methods allows for a diverse and engaging experience.

This not only keeps the practice interesting but also helps seniors discover what resonates most with their unique preferences and needs.

It's essential to view setbacks or challenges as part of the journey and not as failures. Realistic goals in yoga for seniors involve adaptability and a compassionate approach to oneself. If a particular pose or practice proves challenging, modifications can be embraced, and progress can be measured not only in physical achievements but also in the joy and mindfulness cultivated throughout the journey.

Setting realistic goals for seniors in yoga is about fostering a positive and empowering experience. It's a journey that acknowledges the wisdom of the body, celebrates individual progress, and recognizes that the true essence of yoga lies in the ongoing exploration of self-discovery and well-being.

How Yoga Enhances Physical and Mental Well-being

Yoga, a centuries-old practice, serves as a powerful catalyst in promoting the holistic well-being of individuals, profoundly impacting both the physical and mental dimensions of health.

As a versatile discipline, yoga offers a unique blend of physical postures, mindful breathing, and meditation, contributing to a balanced and vibrant life.

Physically, the practice of yoga provides a remarkable avenue for enhancing flexibility, strength, and overall mobility.

Through a series of gentle stretches and poses, individuals engage muscles, tendons, and joints, promoting increased range of motion and reducing stiffness.

This not only aids in daily activities but also mitigates the risk of injury and promotes joint health, particularly crucial for seniors or those managing chronic conditions.

Balance, a fundamental aspect of physical well-being, is honed through various yoga postures. Poses that challenge stability and require focused concentration contribute to improved balance and coordination.

This is particularly valuable for individuals of all ages but holds significant implications for the elderly, reducing the likelihood of falls and enhancing overall physical resilience.

Furthermore, yoga serves as a natural remedy for stress reduction. In a world often characterized by fast-paced living, the meditative and mindful components of yoga offer a sanctuary for tranquility.

By practicing conscious breathing, individuals activate the body's relaxation response, reducing the production of stress hormones and fostering a state of calmness.

This not only alleviates immediate stressors but also cultivates resilience in the face of life's challenges.

The mental benefits of yoga extend beyond stress reduction, encompassing improvements in focus, concentration, and cognitive function. The meditative aspects of yoga, such as mindfulness and awareness, contribute to a heightened sense of presence and mental clarity.

Regular practice has been associated with enhanced cognitive function, memory retention, and a more positive outlook on life.

Moreover, yoga acts as a powerful tool for emotional well-being. The mind-body connection inherent in yoga allows individuals to explore and release stored emotions, promoting a sense of emotional balance and self-awareness.

This aspect is particularly valuable for those managing conditions like anxiety or depression, providing a holistic approach to mental health.

Quality of sleep is intricately linked to overall well-being, and yoga has been shown to contribute to improved sleep patterns. The relaxation techniques employed in yoga, coupled with mindful breathing, help alleviate insomnia and promote restful sleep, leading to enhanced energy levels and better overall health.

As a social activity, group yoga classes foster a sense of community and connection. The shared experience of practicing together creates a supportive environment, reducing feelings of isolation and enhancing overall emotional well-being.

The sense of belonging that arises from participating in a yoga community can be a powerful factor in mental health.

The holistic benefits of yoga extend far beyond physical flexibility and strength. The practice serves as a dynamic means of enhancing mental well-being, offering a comprehensive approach to health that embraces the interconnectedness of the mind and body.

Through the fusion of movement, breath, and mindfulness, yoga becomes a transformative journey toward balance, resilience, and a more profound sense of overall well-being.

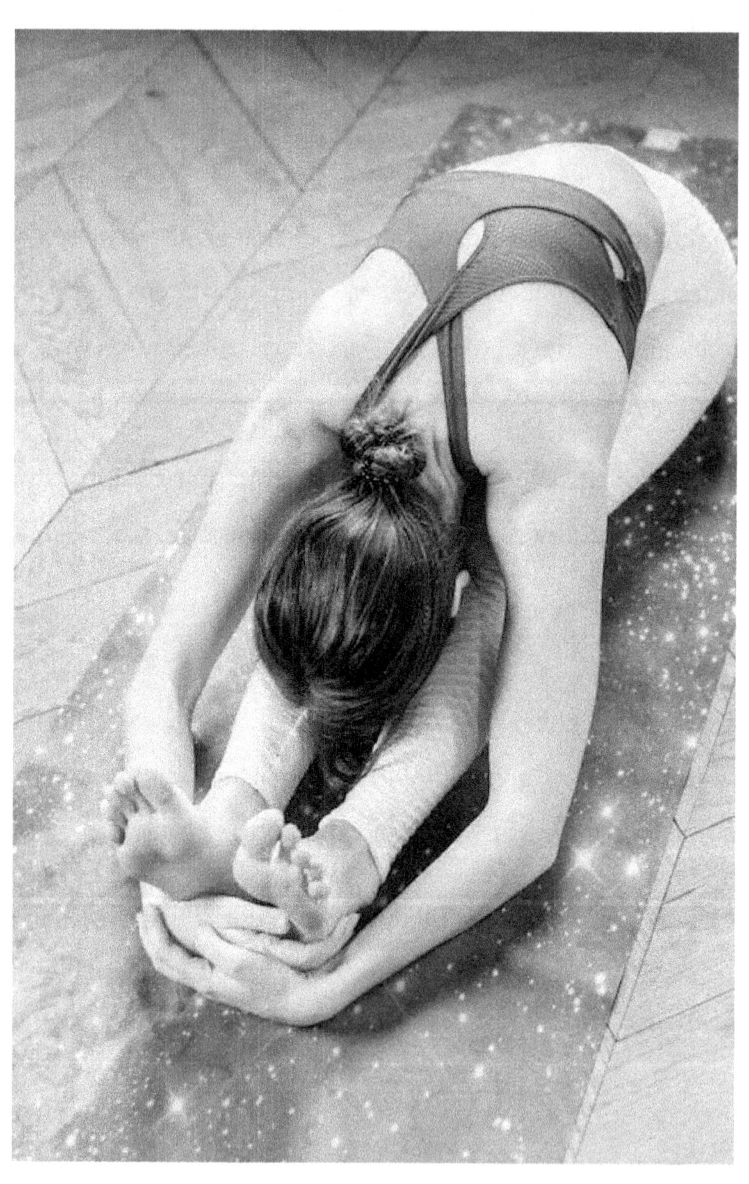

CHAPTER TWO

Seated Yoga Poses for Flexibility and Mobility

Seated yoga poses offer a gentle yet effective approach to enhancing flexibility and mobility, making them particularly beneficial for individuals of all ages and fitness levels.

Whether you're a seasoned yogi or a beginner, incorporating these seated poses into your routine can contribute significantly to overall well-being.

Eexamples of seated yoga poses, their benefits, and instructions on how to practice them:

Sukhasana (Easy Pose):

- Benefits: Grounds and centers the mind, improves posture, and stretches the hips and lower back.
- How to do it: Sit cross-legged, ensuring your spine is straight. Place your hands on your knees with palms facing up or down.

Paschimottanasana (Seated Forward Bend):

- Benefits: Stretches the spine, hamstrings, and lower back; calms the mind.
- How to do it: Sit with legs extended in front. Inhale, lengthen your spine, and exhale as you hinge at the hips, reaching toward your toes.

Baddha Konasana (Bound Angle Pose):

- Benefits: Opens the hips and groin, stimulates abdominal organs, and improves flexibility in the inner thighs.
- How to do it: Sit with the soles of your feet together and knees bent. Hold your feet, lengthen your spine, and gently press your knees toward the floor.

Marjarasana (Cat-Cow Stretch in a Seated Position):

- Benefits: Improves spine flexibility, massages abdominal organs, and promotes a sense of relaxation.
- How to do it: Sit on your shins with hands on your knees. Inhale arching your back (Cow) and exhale rounding your spine (Cat).

Gomukhasana (Cow Face Pose):

- Benefits: Stretches hips, thighs, shoulders, and arms; improves posture.
- How to do it: Stack your knees, bringing one foot beside the opposite hip. Extend the opposite arm overhead, bending the elbow, and reach the other arm behind your back, trying to clasp hands.

Ardha Matsyendrasana (Seated Spinal Twist):

- Benefits: Increases spinal flexibility, stimulates digestion, and stretches the shoulders.
- How to do it: Sit with legs extended, cross one foot over the opposite knee. Twist toward the bent knee, placing the opposite elbow outside the knee.

Dandasana (Staff Pose):

- Benefits: Strengthens the back muscles, improves posture, and stretches the legs.
- How to do it: Sit with legs extended in front, feet flexed. Keep your spine straight, and place your hands on the floor beside your hips.

Upavistha Konasana (Wide-Angle Seated Forward Bend):

- Benefits: Stretches the inner thighs and hamstrings, improves flexibility in the hips.
- How to do it: Sit with legs wide apart. Inhale, lengthen your spine, and exhale as you hinge at the hips, reaching forward.

Janu Sirsasana (Head-to-Knee Forward Bend):

- Benefits: Stretches the spine, hamstrings, and groins; stimulates abdominal organs.
- How to do it: Sit with one leg extended and the other foot against the inner thigh. Inhale, lengthen your spine, and exhale as you fold over the extended leg.

Apanasana (Knees-to-Chest Pose):

- Benefits: Releases tension in the lower back, massages the abdominal organs, and promotes relaxation.
- How to do it: Lie on your back, hug your knees to your chest, and gently rock from side to side.

Vajrasana (Thunderbolt Pose):

- Benefits: Strengthens the pelvic muscles, aids digestion, and improves posture.
- How to do it: Kneel with your buttocks on your heels, keeping your back straight. Place your hands on your thighs or in your lap.

Ankle-to-Knee Pose:

- Benefits: Opens the hips and stretches the outer thighs.
- How to do it: Sit with one knee bent and the ankle resting on the opposite knee. Gently press on the bent knee to deepen the stretch.

Ardha Padmasana (Half Lotus Pose):

- Benefits: Stretches the ankles and knees, improves posture, and enhances hip flexibility.
- How to do it: Sit with one foot on the opposite thigh and the other foot beneath the opposite knee.

Bharadvajasana (Bharadvaja's Twist):

- Benefits: Relieves lower back pain, stretches the spine, and aids in digestion.
- How to do it: Sit with legs extended, then twist to one side, bringing one foot to the outside of the opposite hip.

Malasana (Garland Pose - Seated Variation):

- Benefits: Opens the hips, stretches the ankles, and strengthens the lower back.
- How to do it: Squat down with your feet close together, lower your hips towards the ground, and place your hands in a prayer position.

When practicing these seated yoga poses, remember to listen to your body, breathe deeply, and modify as needed. Regular incorporation of these poses into your routine can lead to improved flexibility, enhanced mobility, and a greater sense of overall well-being.

If you have any existing health concerns, it's advisable to consult with a healthcare professional or a qualified yoga instructor before starting a new yoga practice.

Standing Yoga Poses for Strength and Balance

Standing yoga poses are integral to building strength, stability, and balance. These postures not only enhance physical fitness but also cultivate mindfulness and focus. Incorporating standing poses into your yoga practice can fortify muscles, improve posture, and boost overall well-being.

Examples of standing yoga poses, along with their benefits and instructions on how to perform them:

Tadasana (Mountain Pose):

- Benefits: Improves posture, strengthens thighs and ankles, and enhances awareness of body alignment.
- How to do it: Stand with feet together, arms by your sides, and weight evenly distributed on both feet. Engage thigh muscles and lift your chest.

Virabhadrasana I (Warrior I):

- Benefits: Strengthens legs, opens hips, and builds concentration and endurance.
- How to do it: From Mountain Pose, step one foot back, bend the front knee, and extend arms overhead, palms facing each other.

Virabhadrasana II (Warrior II):

- Benefits: Strengthens legs and core, improves stamina, and opens hips and chest.
- How to do it: Open hips and shoulders to face sideways, arms extended parallel to the floor.

Utthita Trikonasana (Extended Triangle Pose):

- Benefits: Stretches and strengthens the legs, opens the hips, and improves balance.
- How to do it: Stand with legs wide apart, reach one arm down to the ankle of the same side while extending the other arm towards the sky.

Utthita Parsvakonasana (Extended Side Angle Pose):

- Benefits: Strengthens and stretches legs and improves flexibility in the hips and spine.
- How to do it: From Warrior II, lean forward placing the front hand on the ground or a block, and extend the other arm overhead.

Vrksasana (Tree Pose):

- Benefits: Enhances balance, strengthens legs and core, and improves concentration.
- How to do it: Shift weight to one leg, place the sole of the other foot on the inner thigh or calf, and bring hands to the heart center.

Garudasana (Eagle Pose):

- Benefits: Strengthens legs and arms, improves balance, and stretches shoulders and upper back.
- How to do it: Cross one leg over the other, entwine arms, and bend the knees slightly, balancing on one leg.

Utkatasana (Chair Pose):

- Benefits: Strengthens thighs and calves, engages core muscles, and improves posture.
- How to do it: Sit back as if sitting in an imaginary chair, keeping weight in the heels and arms extended overhead.

Anjaneyasana (Low Lunge):

- Benefits: Stretches hip flexors, strengthens thighs, and improves balance.
- How to do it: Step one foot forward into a lunge, lowering the back knee, and raising the arms overhead.

Prasarita Padottanasana (Wide-Legged Forward Bend):

- Benefits: Stretches and strengthens the inner and outer thighs, hamstrings, and lower back.
- How to do it: Stand with legs wide apart, hinge at the hips, and reach hands towards the floor.

Ardha Chandrasana (Half Moon Pose):

- Benefits: Enhances balance, strengthens legs, and opens hips and chest.
- How to do it: From Warrior II, shift weight to front foot, lift back leg, and extend the arm on the same side towards the floor.

Utthita Hasta Padangusthasana (Extended Hand-to-Big-Toe Pose):

- Benefits: Improves balance, strengthens legs and ankles, and stretches hamstrings.
- How to do it: Lift one leg, holding the big toe with the hand of the same side, and extend the leg forward.

Natarajasana (Dancer's Pose):

- Benefits: Enhances balance, strengthens legs and core, and opens the chest and shoulders.
- How to do it: Standing on one leg, reach the opposite hand back to hold the ankle of the lifted foot, extending the other arm forward.

Malasana (Garland Pose - Standing Variation):

- Benefits: Strengthens the legs, opens the hips, and engages the core.
- How to do it: Squat down with feet close together, hands in a prayer position, and elbows pressing against the inner knees.

Hasta Padangusthasana (Hand-to-Big-Toe Pose):

- Benefits: Improves balance, stretches hamstrings, and strengthens legs.
- How to do it: Lift one leg, holding the big toe with the hand of the same side, and extend the leg forward.

When practicing these standing yoga poses, focus on your breath, maintain a steady gaze (drishti), and engage the muscles of your legs and core.

These poses can be adapted for various levels, and modifications can be made to suit your individual needs. Always listen to your body, and if you have any existing health concerns, consult with a healthcare professional or a qualified yoga instructor before starting a new yoga practice.

Modified Sun Salutations for Gentle Warm-ups

Modified Sun Salutations offer a gentle and accessible way to warm up the body, promoting flexibility and circulation. These sequences are particularly beneficial for individuals seeking a milder approach to yoga, including beginners, those with mobility limitations, or individuals looking for a gentle start to their practice. Here, we'll explore a modified Sun Salutation routine that can serve as an effective warm-up, preparing the body for a more extended yoga session.

Basic Sequence:

The following sequence is designed to be gentle and adaptable. It focuses on fluid movements and controlled breathing to warm up the major muscle groups.

1. Mountain Pose (Tadasana):

Stand with feet hip-width apart, arms by your sides, and palms facing forward.

Engage your thighs, lift your chest, and reach your arms overhead.

2. Forward Fold (Uttanasana):

Hinge at your hips, keeping your back straight, and fold forward. Let your hands rest on the floor or shins.

3. Halfway Lift (Ardha Uttanasana):

Lift your upper body halfway, keeping your back straight and parallel to the ground. Extend your spine forward.

4. Low Lunge (Anjaneyasana):

Step one foot back into a lunge position, lowering your back knee. Raise your arms overhead.

5. Downward-Facing Dog (Adho Mukha Svanasana):

Lift your hips, straighten your legs, and form an inverted V-shape. Press your palms into the mat.

6. Plank Pose:

Shift forward into a plank position, aligning your shoulders over your wrists. Engage your core muscles.

7. Knees-Chest-Chin (Ashtanga Namaskara):

Lower your knees, chest, and chin to the mat, keeping your hips elevated.

8. Cobra Pose (Bhujangasana):

Slide forward into a gentle cobra pose, lifting your chest while keeping your lower body on the mat.

9. Downward-Facing Dog (Adho Mukha Svanasana):

Lift your hips back into Downward-Facing Dog.

10. Low Lunge (Anjaneyasana):

Step one foot forward into a low lunge, bringing your arms overhead.

11. Forward Fold (Uttanasana):

Hinge at your hips, fold forward, and bring your hands to the floor or shins.

12. Mountain Pose (Tadasana):

Inhale, engage your thighs, lift your chest, and reach your arms overhead.

Repeat this sequence 3-5 times, flowing with your breath and moving at a comfortable pace.

Benefits of Modified Sun Salutations:

- Gentle Warm-up: The sequence gradually warms up the entire body, promoting flexibility in the spine, shoulders, and hips.
- Improved Circulation: Controlled breathing enhances blood flow, delivering oxygen to muscles and joints.
- Enhanced Mobility: Each movement targets different muscle groups, encouraging increased range of motion.
- Mind-Body Connection: Focusing on breath and movement cultivates mindfulness, promoting a sense of calmness.

Additional Seated Yoga Poses for Warm-ups:

While the above sequence predominantly involves standing and transitioning poses, integrating seated poses can provide a well-rounded warm-up routine. Here are a few seated poses with their benefits:

Easy Pose (Sukhasana):

- Benefits: Grounds and centers the mind, opens hips.
- How to do it: Sit cross-legged with a straight spine.

Seated Forward Bend (Paschimottanasana):

- ➢ Benefits: Stretches the spine, hamstrings, and lower back.
- ➢ How to do it: Sit with legs extended, hinge at the hips, and reach toward your toes.

Butterfly Pose (Baddha Konasana):

- ➢ Benefits: Opens the hips and groin.
- ➢ How to do it: Sit with the soles of your feet together, knees bent outward.

Seated Twist (Ardha Matsyendrasana):

- ➢ Benefits: Improves spinal flexibility, stimulates digestion.
- ➢ How to do it: Sit with one leg extended, cross the other leg over, and twist.

Cow Face Pose (Gomukhasana):

- ➢ Benefits: Stretches hips, thighs, and shoulders.
- ➢ How to do it: Stack one knee over the other and bring arms into a bind.

Staff Pose (Dandasana):

- ➤ Benefits: Strengthens the back muscles, improves posture.
- ➤ How to do it: Sit with legs extended, keeping the spine straight.

Seated Side Stretch (Parsva Sukhasana):

- ➤ Benefits: Stretches the sides of the body.
- ➤ How to do it: Sit cross-legged, reach one arm overhead, and lean to the side.

Wide-Angle Seated Forward Bend (Upavistha Konasana):

- ➤ Benefits: Stretches the inner thighs and hamstrings.
- ➤ How to do it: Sit with legs wide apart, hinge at the hips, and reach forward.

Seated Cat-Cow (Marjarasana):

- ➤ Benefits: Improves spine flexibility.
- ➤ How to do it: Sit with hands on knees, arch and round the spine.

Seated Pigeon Pose (Eka Pada Rajakapotasana):

> ➢ Benefits: Opens hips and stretches the outer thighs.

> ➢ How to do it: Cross one ankle over the opposite knee and gently press on the bent knee.

Seated Camel Pose (Ustrasana):

> ➢ Benefits: Stretches the front of the body.

> ➢ How to do it: Kneel with hips over knees, lift the chest, and reach back.

Seated Mountain Pose (Parvatasana):

> ➢ Benefits: Strengthens the arms and engages the core.

> ➢ How to do it: Sit with legs extended, reach arms overhead, and interlace fingers.

Seated Twist (Ardha Matsyendrasana):

> ➢ Benefits: Increases spinal flexibility, stimulates digestion.

> ➢ How to do it: Sit with one leg extended, cross the other leg over, and twist.

Seated Garland Pose (Malasana):

> ➢ Benefits: Strengthens the legs, opens the hips.

> How to do it: Squat down with feet close together, elbows pressing against the inner knees.

Seated Forward Bend (Paschimottanasana):

> Benefits: Stretches the spine, hamstrings, and lower back.

> How to do it: Sit with legs extended, hinge at the hips, and reach toward your toes.

Integrating these seated poses with modified Sun Salutations creates a well-rounded warm-up routine suitable for individuals of various fitness levels and needs.

As always, listen to your body, breathe deeply, and modify the poses as necessary. If you have any existing health concerns, consult with a healthcare professional or a qualified yoga instructor before starting a new yoga practice.

Incorporating Props for Support and Comfort

In the world of yoga, the use of props adds a dimension of support and comfort, transforming the practice into a personalized and adaptable experience. Props, ranging from blocks and straps to blankets and bolsters, serve as invaluable tools for practitioners of all levels, aiding in alignment, stability, and relaxation. Incorporating props into yoga practice not only enhances comfort but also allows individuals to explore the depths of each pose safely and effectively.

One of the primary benefits of using props is the support they offer in achieving proper alignment. Whether you're a beginner refining your postures or an experienced practitioner working on advanced poses, props assist in finding the optimal position for your body.

For instance, blocks can be strategically placed under hands or feet to modify the height and reach in various poses, ensuring that the body is aligned correctly without strain.

Props also play a crucial role in making yoga accessible for individuals with physical limitations or injuries. For those with tight muscles or limited flexibility, straps can be employed to extend reach in stretches, gradually improving range of motion over time.

This inclusivity fosters an environment where yoga becomes a practice for everyone, regardless of their physical condition, age, or level of experience.

In restorative yoga practices, props become the key to deep relaxation. Blankets and bolsters support the body in restful poses, promoting a sense of ease and surrender.

Restorative poses, such as supported savasana or reclining bound angle pose, allow practitioners to experience profound relaxation, releasing tension and calming the nervous system. This nurturing aspect of prop-supported yoga is particularly beneficial for stress reduction and mental well-being.

In addition to providing physical support, props can intensify the challenge in certain poses. For instance, a block can be placed between the thighs in chair pose, adding resistance and engaging inner thigh muscles more actively.

This versatility makes props invaluable tools for both beginners easing into the practice and advanced practitioners seeking to deepen their experience.

The versatility of props extends to therapeutic applications as well. Individuals recovering from injuries or dealing with chronic conditions can use props to adapt poses to their unique needs.

A chair, for example, can provide support for individuals with balance issues, allowing them to safely practice standing poses with stability.

To incorporate props into your yoga practice, it's essential to understand their roles in different poses. Blocks can assist in standing poses and seated stretches, while straps are excellent for enhancing flexibility in forward bends and leg stretches. Blankets and bolsters are ideal for restorative poses and deep relaxation.

As a general principle, props should be used to enhance the yoga experience, not as a crutch. They provide the necessary assistance to gradually progress in the practice, building strength, flexibility, and mindfulness over time.

The integration of props into yoga practice is a testament to the adaptability and inclusivity of this ancient discipline.

Whether you're seeking support, relaxation, or an extra challenge, props offer a myriad of possibilities to tailor your practice to your unique needs.

As you explore the world of yoga with props, you embark on a journey of self-discovery, embracing the transformative power of a practice that is both accessible and infinitely enriching.

Guided Meditation for Stress Reduction

Guided meditation stands as a powerful tool in the arsenal against stress, offering a structured and calming approach to navigate the complexities of the mind.

In a world inundated with constant stimuli, guided meditation provides a respite, guiding individuals through a journey of self-reflection and tranquility. This practice, rooted in mindfulness and intentionality, proves particularly effective in stress reduction, cultivating a state of inner calm and resilience.

Central to guided meditation is the calming influence of a narrator or guide, whether in person or through a recorded session. The guide leads participants through a series of mental images, breath awareness, and relaxation techniques, creating a focused and serene mental environment.

The guided nature of the meditation eliminates the need for individuals to structure their own practice, making it accessible and appealing to those new to meditation.

One of the primary benefits of guided meditation for stress reduction is its ability to redirect the mind's attention away from stressors and into the present moment. The guided instructions encourage participants to anchor their awareness to the breath or other sensory experiences, creating a mental refuge from the chaos of daily life.

This shift in focus allows individuals to detach from the overwhelming thoughts associated with stress, fostering a sense of mental clarity and calm.

Breath awareness is a cornerstone of many guided meditations, acting as a powerful tool to regulate the nervous system and induce a relaxation response.

By guiding participants to observe and deepen their breath, these sessions activate the parasympathetic nervous system, countering the effects of the stress-inducing sympathetic nervous system.

This intentional focus on the breath becomes a steady anchor, providing individuals with a tangible point of concentration amid life's storms.

Visualization is another key component of guided meditation, transporting individuals to mental landscapes that evoke peace and tranquility. Whether envisioning a serene beach, a lush forest, or a mountain retreat, these visualizations engage the imagination, creating a mental sanctuary.

This mental escapade not only reduces stress in the moment but also equips individuals with a visualization tool they can employ independently in times of heightened stress.

Guided meditation often incorporates body scan techniques, encouraging a mindful exploration of physical sensations. This process of turning attention inward allows individuals to identify and release tension held in different parts of the body, promoting a holistic sense of relaxation.

As the body releases physical stress, the mind follows suit, creating a harmonious and integrated experience of well-being.

Consistency is key to reaping the full benefits of guided meditation for stress reduction. Regular practice conditions the mind to respond more adaptively to stressors, fostering resilience and an enhanced ability to maintain composure in challenging situations. Over time, the skills cultivated in guided meditation become an integral part of an individual's stress management toolkit.

In essence, guided meditation for stress reduction serves as a structured pathway to inner peace. By immersing individuals in a guided journey of breath awareness, visualization, and body scan, this practice becomes a sanctuary for the mind, offering respite from the demands of a hectic world.

As participants embrace the guided meditation experience, they unlock the transformative potential of mindfulness, paving the way to a more balanced and stress-resilient life.

Breathing Exercises to Enhance Lung Capacity

Breathing exercises play a pivotal role in optimizing lung capacity, promoting respiratory health, and fostering overall well-being. As an integral aspect of a holistic approach to health, these exercises go beyond simply providing oxygen to the body; they enhance the efficiency and strength of the respiratory system.

Whether practiced for general wellness, athletic performance, or managing respiratory conditions, intentional breathing exercises empower individuals to harness the full potential of their lungs.

Diaphragmatic Breathing:

Diaphragmatic breathing, also known as abdominal or deep breathing, is a fundamental exercise to enhance lung capacity. It involves the contraction and relaxation of the diaphragm, allowing the lungs to fill with air more efficiently.

To practice diaphragmatic breathing, sit or lie down comfortably, place one hand on the chest and the other on the abdomen. Inhale deeply through the nose, feeling the abdomen rise, and exhale slowly through pursed lips.

Pursed Lip Breathing:

This technique helps improve lung function by keeping airways open longer, preventing the collapse of small air passages. Inhale slowly through the nose for two counts, and exhale through pursed lips for four counts. Pursed lip breathing promotes the release of trapped air in the lungs and reduces the work of breathing.

Box Breathing (Square Breathing):

Box breathing is a simple yet effective exercise that enhances lung capacity and promotes relaxation.

Inhale through the nose for a count of four, hold the breath for four counts, exhale through the mouth for four counts, and then pause for another four counts before beginning the next cycle.

This rhythmic pattern maximizes oxygen intake while encouraging mental focus and calming the nervous system.

Alternate Nostril Breathing (Nadi Shodhana):

Nadi Shodhana, a yogic breathing technique, helps balance the flow of energy in the body and improves lung capacity.

Sit comfortably, use the thumb and ring finger to alternately close one nostril while inhaling and exhaling through the other.

This method not only enhances respiratory function but also brings a sense of balance and calmness.

Resistance Breathing:

Incorporating resistance into breathing exercises can strengthen respiratory muscles and increase lung capacity.

Using a handheld device designed for respiratory muscle training, inhale against resistance, and then exhale slowly. This resistance challenges the lungs, promoting greater strength and endurance over time.

Belly Breathing with Visualization:

Combine diaphragmatic breathing with visualization to enhance the effectiveness of the exercise. Inhale deeply, imagining your lungs filling with fresh, invigorating air.

As you exhale, visualize releasing any tension or stale air. This technique not only improves lung capacity but also fosters a mindful connection between breath and visualization.

Humming Bee Breath (Bhramari Pranayama):

Bhramari pranayama involves producing a humming sound during exhalation, which can strengthen the respiratory muscles and improve airflow. Sit comfortably, close your eyes, and inhale deeply.

Exhale while making a humming sound like a bee. This practice helps reduce stress, enhance lung capacity, and promote a sense of calm.

Regular practice of these breathing exercises not only improves lung capacity but also enhances respiratory efficiency, increases oxygen supply to the body, and reduces stress.

It's essential to approach these exercises mindfully and consistently integrate them into your routine for optimal benefits. Individuals with pre-existing respiratory conditions should consult with healthcare professionals or respiratory therapists before beginning new breathing exercises.

Chair Yoga for Relaxation and Mindful Awareness

Chair yoga provides a gentle yet powerful avenue for relaxation and mindful awareness, making the benefits of yoga accessible to individuals with varying levels of mobility.

As a versatile practice, chair yoga adapts traditional yoga poses to a seated or supported position, allowing participants to experience the transformative effects of yoga without the need for a mat or complex movements. This form of yoga is particularly well-suited for those with limited mobility, seniors, or anyone seeking a calming practice that nurtures both the body and mind.

Mindful Awareness in Chair Yoga:

Chair yoga places a strong emphasis on mindful awareness, inviting practitioners to cultivate a deep connection between breath, movement, and the present moment.

By focusing on the sensations in the body, the rhythm of the breath, and the subtleties of movement, participants can develop a heightened sense of mindfulness. This intentional awareness not only enhances the yoga experience but also acts as a gateway to stress reduction and mental tranquility.

Adapted Poses for Relaxation:

Chair yoga incorporates a variety of adapted poses that promote relaxation and flexibility. Seated forward bends, gentle twists, and modified stretches allow participants to release tension held in the neck, shoulders, and spine. These poses are designed to be accessible to individuals of all fitness levels, providing a safe and supportive environment for relaxation.

Breath-Centered Practices:

Chair yoga often integrates breath-centered practices to enhance relaxation and mindful awareness.

Techniques such as diaphragmatic breathing, where emphasis is placed on deep inhalations and exhalations, serve to activate the body's relaxation response.

The rhythmic flow of breath becomes a focal point, promoting a sense of calmness and grounding.

Seated Meditation and Mindful Movement:

The practice of seated meditation is seamlessly woven into chair yoga sessions, fostering a contemplative atmosphere.

Participants are guided to bring attention to the present moment, anchoring themselves in the sensations of the breath and the gentle movements of the body.

This integration of meditation into chair yoga contributes to stress reduction, improved concentration, and an overall sense of well-being.

Gentle Stretching and Joint Mobility:

Chair yoga incorporates gentle stretching and joint mobility exercises to enhance flexibility and release tension. By encouraging fluid movements within the limitations of a seated position, individuals can experience the benefits of increased circulation, improved range of motion, and a sense of revitalization.

Accessible Mindfulness Practices:

Chair yoga makes mindfulness practices accessible to a broader audience, including those who may face physical limitations.

Mindful awareness is cultivated not only through physical postures but also through guided imagery, breath awareness, and visualization. These accessible techniques empower individuals to develop a mindful presence in their daily lives beyond the yoga session.

Community and Social Connection:

Chair yoga often takes place in group settings, fostering a sense of community and social connection. The shared experience of practicing mindful awareness in a supportive group setting can contribute to a positive and uplifting atmosphere. This sense of belonging and shared intention enhances the overall mental well-being of participants.

CHAPTER THREE

Progressive Muscle Relaxation for Seniors

Progressive Muscle Relaxation (PMR) stands out as an effective and accessible relaxation technique for seniors, offering a systematic approach to releasing physical tension and promoting overall well-being.

Tailored to suit the needs of older adults, PMR provides a gentle yet impactful way to alleviate stress, improve sleep, and enhance the mind-body connection.

This evidence-based practice is particularly beneficial for seniors looking to cultivate a greater sense of relaxation and comfort in their daily lives.

Understanding Progressive Muscle Relaxation:

PMR, developed by physician Edmund Jacobson in the 1920s, involves the intentional tensing and subsequent relaxation of muscle groups.

The practice systematically moves through different areas of the body, encouraging individuals to become more aware of physical sensations and promoting a deep state of relaxation.

This approach makes PMR a valuable tool for seniors seeking to manage stress, reduce anxiety, and enhance their overall quality of life.

Adaptations for Seniors:

One of the strengths of PMR is its adaptability. For seniors, modifications can be made to suit individual abilities and comfort levels.

The practice can be done seated or lying down, allowing seniors to choose a position that feels most comfortable. Additionally, adjustments to the duration of muscle tensing and relaxation can be made to accommodate the unique needs of older adults.

Enhanced Mind-Body Connection:

PMR fosters a heightened awareness of the mind-body connection, encouraging seniors to tune into the physical sensations of each muscle group.

This increased awareness helps individuals identify and release tension stored in the body, promoting a sense of relaxation and ease.

As seniors become more attuned to their bodies, they often experience a greater sense of control over their stress responses.

Stress Reduction and Improved Sleep:

Seniors often face stressors related to health, family, and lifestyle changes. PMR serves as a powerful tool to counteract the effects of stress, triggering the relaxation response and promoting a sense of calm.

The practice has also been associated with improved sleep quality, which is particularly beneficial for seniors who may face challenges with sleep disorders or insomnia.

Increased Mobility and Flexibility:

The intentional engagement and release of muscle groups in PMR contribute to improved mobility and flexibility. For seniors, maintaining and enhancing physical function is crucial for maintaining independence and overall well-being.

Regular practice of PMR can complement other physical activities, helping to address issues related to muscle stiffness and joint discomfort.

Community and Social Benefits:

While PMR is often practiced individually, it can also be integrated into group settings, providing a shared experience for seniors.

Group sessions foster a sense of community and social connection, contributing to overall mental and emotional well-being.

The camaraderie within a group can create a supportive environment where seniors feel encouraged to prioritize their relaxation and self-care.

Building Resilience and Coping Skills:

Seniors may face various stressors, including health concerns and life transitions. PMR equips individuals with valuable coping skills and resilience-building techniques.

By incorporating PMR into their routine, seniors can develop a proactive approach to stress management, enhancing their ability to navigate challenges and transitions with greater ease.

Progressive Muscle Relaxation emerges as a valuable and accessible practice for seniors, offering a pathway to stress reduction, improved sleep, and enhanced well-being.

The adaptability of PMR makes it suitable for individuals of varying abilities, allowing seniors to experience the benefits of intentional muscle relaxation in a way that suits their unique needs.

As seniors incorporate PMR into their daily routines, they not only release physical tension but also cultivate a deeper connection between the body and mind, fostering a greater sense of peace and resilience.

Designing a Customized Routine for Individual Needs

Designing a customized routine tailored to individual needs is a key aspect of promoting overall well-being and achieving personal health goals.

Whether focusing on physical fitness, mental well-being, or a combination of both, a personalized routine ensures that individuals address their unique strengths, challenges, and preferences. Here are essential considerations for creating a customized routine that aligns with individual needs:

Assessment of Personal Goals:

The first step in designing a customized routine is a thorough assessment of personal goals. Individuals need to identify specific objectives, whether it's improving physical fitness, managing stress, enhancing flexibility, or achieving a balance between different aspects of well-being.

Clear and realistic goals serve as the foundation for building a routine that is both meaningful and achievable.

Understanding Physical and Mental Capabilities:

Taking stock of physical and mental capabilities is crucial. Consider factors such as current fitness level, health conditions, flexibility, and mental resilience.

This self-awareness allows individuals to tailor their routine to match their current capacities while gradually challenging themselves for improvement.

Incorporating Variety and Enjoyment:

A customized routine should be diverse and enjoyable to ensure sustained engagement. Incorporating a mix of activities, such as cardiovascular exercises, strength training, flexibility work, and mindfulness practices, adds variety to the routine.

Including activities that individuals genuinely enjoy increases the likelihood of sticking with the routine over the long term.

Setting Realistic and Incremental Milestones:

Realistic and incremental milestones play a pivotal role in maintaining motivation and tracking progress. Break larger goals into smaller, achievable steps.

Celebrating these milestones fosters a sense of accomplishment and encourages individuals to stay committed to their routine.

Flexibility for Lifestyle and Schedule:

A customized routine must be flexible and adaptable to fit into one's lifestyle and schedule. Considerations such as work commitments, family responsibilities, and personal preferences are essential. A routine that can be seamlessly integrated into daily life increases the likelihood of consistency.

Balancing Physical and Mental Well-being:

Recognizing the interconnectedness of physical and mental well-being is vital.

A holistic routine addresses both aspects, incorporating not only physical exercises but also mindfulness practices, relaxation techniques, and activities that promote mental resilience. Balancing these elements contributes to overall health and a sense of harmony.

Consultation with Professionals:

Seeking guidance from healthcare professionals, fitness trainers, or mental health experts can provide valuable insights.

Professionals can help tailor a routine that aligns with individual needs, taking into account any health concerns or specific requirements. This consultation ensures that the routine is safe, effective, and aligned with personal goals.

Regular Monitoring and Adjustments:

A customized routine is not static; it requires regular monitoring and adjustments. Individuals should pay attention to how their body and mind respond to the routine, making modifications as needed. Adapting the routine based on evolving needs ensures continuous progress and prevents plateaus.

Mindful Self-Care Practices:

Incorporating mindful self-care practices is essential for overall well-being. This may include activities such as meditation, deep breathing exercises, or engaging in hobbies that bring joy and relaxation. Mindful self-care contributes to mental clarity, emotional resilience, and a positive outlook.

Social Support and Accountability:

Building a routine with social support and accountability enhances the likelihood of success. Whether through workout partners, support groups, or sharing progress with friends and family, having a support system creates a positive environment that reinforces commitment.

Creating a Safe and Comfortable Yoga Space at Home

Creating a safe and comfortable yoga space at home is essential for cultivating a harmonious environment that supports your practice.

Whether you're a seasoned yogi or just starting your journey, the space you practice in can significantly impact your overall experience.

Here are key considerations for establishing a serene and safe yoga haven within the confines of your home:

Selecting the Right Space:

Begin by identifying a dedicated area in your home for yoga. Ideally, choose a quiet and clutter-free space where you can move freely without disruptions.

Whether it's a spare room, a corner in your living room, or even a spot on your balcony, the key is to find a space that feels inviting and can be easily maintained.

Clearing Clutter and Distractions:

A clutter-free space is conducive to a focused and serene yoga practice. Clear the area of unnecessary items, ensuring that you have enough room to stretch and move without hindrance.

Minimize distractions by turning off electronic devices and creating a tranquil ambiance with soft lighting and calming colors.

Investing in Quality Yoga Props:

Yoga props enhance your practice and contribute to a safe environment. Invest in a good-quality yoga mat that provides sufficient cushioning and grip.

Depending on your practice, consider props such as blocks, straps, and bolsters. These props assist in maintaining proper alignment and offer support during various poses.

Ensuring Adequate Ventilation:

Good air circulation is crucial for a comfortable practice. Ensure that the yoga space is well-ventilated, allowing fresh air to flow freely.

Open windows or doors if possible, or use a fan to maintain a pleasant temperature. A well-ventilated space helps create an atmosphere that supports deep breathing and relaxation.

Creating a Calming Atmosphere:

Infuse your yoga space with elements that promote tranquility. Consider incorporating soft lighting, such as lamps or candles, to create a warm and calming ambiance.

Choose colors that evoke a sense of serenity, such as soothing blues or earthy tones. Play gentle music or nature sounds to enhance the overall atmosphere.

Establishing Proper Lighting:

Natural light can greatly enhance your practice, so if possible, choose a space with ample daylight.

If practicing in the evening or in a room with limited natural light, incorporate adjustable lighting to create the right mood.

Soft, diffused lighting is preferable, avoiding harsh or glaring lights that can be distracting.

Ensuring a Level and Stable Surface:

A level and stable surface are essential for a safe yoga practice. Ensure that your yoga mat is placed on a flat, non-slippery surface to prevent any accidents or injuries.

If practicing on a carpet, make sure it provides a stable foundation. A level surface contributes to proper alignment and stability during poses.

Personalizing the Space with Inspiration:

Personalize your yoga space with items that inspire and uplift you. This could include meaningful artwork, motivational quotes, or symbols that hold significance to your practice.

Creating a space that resonates with positive energy contributes to a sense of connection and purpose during your yoga sessions.

Prioritizing Safety and Alignment:

Safety should be a top priority in your yoga space. Ensure that the floor is free of hazards, such as loose rugs or slippery surfaces. Position yourself away from furniture or sharp objects that may pose a risk during certain poses.

Pay attention to proper alignment to prevent strain or injury during your practice.

Establishing Consistent Rituals:

Create a sense of ritual around your yoga practice. This could involve lighting a candle, setting an intention, or incorporating a brief meditation before and after your session. Consistent rituals signal to your mind that it's time to transition into a focused and mindful practice.

By incorporating these considerations into your home yoga space, you create an environment that nurtures your practice and supports your overall well-being.

A safe and comfortable space encourages regularity, allowing you to fully immerse yourself in the transformative benefits of yoga within the sanctuary of your home.

Integrating Yoga into Daily Activities

Integrating yoga into daily activities is a holistic approach to infuse mindfulness, flexibility, and tranquility into the rhythm of your life. While dedicating time to a formal yoga practice is valuable, weaving yogic principles and movements into everyday tasks enhances overall well-being.

Here's how you can seamlessly incorporate yoga into your daily routine:

1. Mindful Breathing in Daily Commutes:

Transform your daily commute into a mindful journey. While driving, waiting for public transport, or even walking, focus on your breath.

Practice deep, intentional inhales and exhales, cultivating a sense of calmness amid the hustle and bustle. Mindful breathing during your commute can create a peaceful transition between home and work.

2. Desk Yoga for Work Breaks:

Counteract the sedentary nature of desk work with simple desk yoga stretches. Incorporate seated stretches, wrist rotations, neck stretches, and shoulder rolls to release tension. These mini-yoga breaks not only promote physical flexibility but also rejuvenate the mind, enhancing focus and productivity.

3. Yoga Poses During Daily Chores:

Turn daily chores into an opportunity for gentle stretching.

While standing in line or waiting for your coffee to brew, practice standing yoga poses like Tadasana (Mountain Pose) to improve posture and balance.

Integrate forward folds or lunges while picking up items from the floor, transforming routine activities into mini yoga sequences.

4. Mindful Eating Practices:

Bring mindfulness to your meals by incorporating yogic principles into your eating habits. Before meals, take a moment to express gratitude. Chew your food slowly, savoring each bite.

This mindful approach to eating aligns with yoga's emphasis on being present and fosters a healthier relationship with food.

5. Yoga Nidra Before Bed:

Integrate yoga into your bedtime routine with Yoga Nidra, a guided meditation for deep relaxation. Lie down comfortably before sleep and follow a Yoga Nidra recording. This practice not only helps in winding down but also promotes restful sleep and mental rejuvenation.

6. Standing Poses While Waiting:

Utilize waiting time to practice standing yoga poses discreetly. Whether waiting for an elevator or in a queue, engage your muscles by standing tall in Mountain Pose or balancing on one leg in Tree Pose.

These subtle poses enhance stability, strengthen your legs, and cultivate mindfulness in everyday situations.

7. Breathing Exercises in Stressful Moments:

When faced with stressful situations, deploy yogic breathing techniques. Take a moment to practice deep diaphragmatic breaths, inhaling slowly through your nose and exhaling through pursed lips. This calms the nervous system, reducing stress and promoting a centered mindset.

8. Yoga Stretches During Screen Time:

Combat the effects of prolonged screen time by incorporating seated yoga stretches. While watching TV or working on the computer, practice seated forward folds, neck stretches, and wrist exercises. These stretches alleviate tension, improve circulation, and counteract the impact of extended periods of sitting.

9. Mindful Walking for Exercise:

Transform your daily walk into a mindful practice. Focus on your breath, observe your surroundings, and engage in a walking meditation.

Pay attention to each step, fostering a sense of presence and grounding. This mindful approach turns a simple walk into a holistic movement experience.

10. Yoga-Inspired Mindfulness in Daily Interactions:

Extend yogic principles into your interactions with others. Practice active listening, speak mindfully, and approach conversations with compassion.

Cultivating mindfulness in your communication fosters positive connections and aligns with yoga's emphasis on kindness and understanding.

By integrating yoga into your daily activities, you infuse mindfulness and movement into your routine, promoting physical and mental well-being.

These seamless incorporations of yoga principles enhance the quality of your daily life, transforming ordinary moments into opportunities for self-care and self-awareness.

Connecting with Yoga Communities and Classes for Seniors

Connecting with yoga communities and classes is a wonderful way for seniors to embark on a journey of holistic well-being.

Engaging in a supportive and like-minded community provides numerous physical, mental, and social benefits. Here's why and how seniors can connect with yoga communities and classes:

1. Social Connection and Support:

Yoga classes offer seniors a sense of community and social connection.

Joining a group of individuals who share an interest in yoga creates a supportive environment. This sense of belonging can be especially valuable for seniors, fostering friendships, and combating feelings of isolation.

2. Tailored Instruction for Seniors:

Attending yoga classes specifically designed for seniors ensures that the practice is adapted to individual needs and limitations.

Instructors with expertise in senior yoga can guide participants through poses and sequences that enhance flexibility, balance, and overall well-being while taking into account any existing health concerns.

3. Physical Health and Well-being:

Yoga classes provide a structured approach to improving physical health for seniors. Gentle movements, stretching, and strengthening exercises contribute to enhanced flexibility, joint mobility, and muscle tone.

Regular attendance can alleviate stiffness, reduce the risk of falls, and support overall physical well-being.

4. Mental Well-being and Stress Reduction:

Yoga is renowned for its positive impact on mental health, and seniors can benefit significantly. Mindful breathing, meditation, and relaxation techniques incorporated in classes contribute to stress reduction, improved mood, and increased mental clarity. Seniors often find that yoga provides a calming space for self-reflection and emotional well-being.

5. Accessible Yoga for All Abilities:

Yoga classes for seniors are designed to be accessible to individuals with varying abilities. Inclusive instruction ensures that everyone, regardless of fitness level or mobility, can participate.

Modified poses and the use of props create an inclusive environment where seniors can feel comfortable and confident in their practice.

6. Community Events and Gatherings:

Many yoga communities organize events and gatherings beyond regular classes. Seniors can participate in workshops, seminars, or social activities organized by the yoga community. These events provide additional opportunities for learning, socializing, and deepening their connection with the yoga community.

7. Mindful Aging and Self-Care:

Yoga classes for seniors often emphasize mindful aging and self-care practices.

Instructors guide participants in embracing the aging process with grace, cultivating self-compassion, and fostering a positive attitude towards their bodies.

These classes go beyond physical postures, incorporating wisdom and mindfulness tailored to the unique experiences of seniors.

8. Flexibility in Class Formats:

Yoga communities offer flexibility in class formats, allowing seniors to choose sessions that align with their preferences and schedules. Whether it's gentle yoga, chair yoga, or restorative yoga, seniors can explore different class styles to

find what suits them best. The variety of options ensures that individuals can adapt their practice based on their energy levels, physical condition, and personal preferences.

9. Encouraging Consistency and Routine:

Being part of a yoga community encourages consistency and routine in practice. Seniors can establish a regular schedule for attending classes, providing a structured and beneficial routine for physical and mental well-being.

Consistent practice is key to experiencing the full range of benefits that yoga offers.

10. Inspiration and Motivation:

Connecting with a yoga community provides seniors with inspiration and motivation. Witnessing the progress and achievements of fellow practitioners, sharing experiences, and celebrating milestones fosters a positive and uplifting atmosphere. This mutual encouragement can be a powerful motivator for seniors to stay committed to their yoga practice.

11. Online Options for Accessibility:

For seniors who may prefer practicing from the comfort of their homes, or those with mobility constraints, many yoga communities offer online classes.

Virtual platforms provide accessibility, allowing seniors to join classes from anywhere, at any time. Online options ensure that yoga remains within reach for those who may face challenges in attending in-person sessions.

12. Adaptable and Supportive Instructors:

Instructors within senior yoga communities are often experienced and attuned to the unique needs of older adults. They provide guidance, encouragement, and adjustments tailored to each individual.

The adaptability and support offered by knowledgeable instructors create a safe and nurturing environment for seniors to explore and deepen their yoga practice.

Connecting with yoga communities and classes is a transformative experience for seniors, offering a holistic approach to well-being.

From the physical benefits of improved flexibility and balance to the mental advantages of stress reduction and mindfulness, participating in yoga classes fosters a sense of community, support, and joy.

Seniors can embark on this enriching journey, discovering the profound impact that yoga can have on their overall health and quality of life.

CONCLUSION

Yoga emerges as a beacon of holistic well-being for seniors, offering a myriad of physical, mental, and social benefits. As individuals gracefully navigate the golden years, the practice of yoga becomes a transformative ally, promoting flexibility, strength, and balance.

The gentle yet powerful nature of senior-specific yoga classes ensures that the practice is accessible to all, regardless of age or fitness level.

The physical advantages of yoga for seniors extend beyond the mat, permeating daily activities and enhancing overall mobility. From improved joint health to increased muscle tone, yoga fosters resilience in the face of age-related challenges.

Moreover, the mindful incorporation of breathwork and meditation facilitates stress reduction, contributing to a positive outlook and emotional well-being.

The sense of community forged within yoga classes for seniors is equally vital. Beyond the physical postures, the shared experiences, encouragement, and camaraderie create a supportive environment. This community-driven approach not only combats feelings of isolation but also fosters a collective journey toward wellness.

Yoga's adaptability shines through, providing tailored practices such as chair yoga or gentle flows that accommodate varying abilities. Instructors with expertise in senior yoga guide practitioners with care, ensuring a safe and enjoyable exploration of movement and mindfulness.

As seniors embrace the principles of yoga, they not only enhance their physical health but also embark on a journey of self-discovery and mindful aging.

The regularity and routine instilled by yoga classes contribute to a sustained commitment to well-being, proving that it's never too late to cultivate a healthier, more balanced life.

In essence, yoga for seniors transcends the physical postures; it becomes a source of inspiration, resilience, and joy. From the first breath on the mat to the moments of reflection and community connection, yoga becomes a timeless companion on the path to aging gracefully and embracing the full spectrum of well-being in one's later years.